Pocket PCOS

A Quick and Practical Guide to Polycystic Ovary Syndrome with Personal Testimonies

Christopher Hearn and
Shahab S. Minassian, M.D.

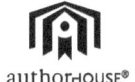

authorHOUSE®

AuthorHouse™
1663 Liberty Drive, Suite 200
Bloomington, IN 47403
www.authorhouse.com
Phone: 1-800-839-8640

First published by AuthorHouse 6/27/2008

ISBN: 978-1-4343-5714-4 (sc)

Printed in the United States of America
Bloomington, Indiana

This book is printed on acid-free paper.

Cover photo taken by Christopher Hearn.

Dedications

I dedicate this book to my lovely wife, who has long suffered with Polycystic Ovary Syndrome. Like many women who have this disease, she has struggled valiantly to live a normal life in the midst of very abnormal circumstances. May all the women who read this book find strength, hope and encouragement to rise above the disease and be their true selves.

Christopher Hearn

This book is dedicated to my teacher and friend, Chung H. Wu, M.D., who laid the foundation for my knowledge in the syndrome, and taught me to think beyond the traditional and accepted.

Shahab S. Minassian, M.D.

Foreword

The polycystic ovary (or ovarian) syndrome, most commonly known by its acronym PCOS, was first described in 1935, and is now recognized to affect as many as one in every ten to twelve women of reproductive age.

PCOS is a syndrome, that is, a collection of signs and features, and no single test is sufficient to diagnose PCOS. Women with PCOS frequently have excess male hormones, which can lead to excess facial and body hair growth, acne, and even scalp hair thinning. They also almost always have irregular ovulation, which leads to irregular menstrual cycles and infertility. And because many women with PCOS are overweight and have insulin resistance (where the hormone insulin, which regulates blood sugar levels, among other things, has a hard time working properly) they tend to have a greater risk for diabetes and heart disease.

Many women with PCOS suffer significantly, often made worse because some physicians, and even the patients themselves, do not recognize the presence of the disorder, and do not know how to diagnose it or how to best treat it.

To help patients with PCOS understand their disorder, Mr. Christopher Hearn and Dr. Shahab S. Minassian have written a short monograph on PCOS. It will be very useful for many patients, whether new to the disorder or having experienced PCOS for many years.

Mr. Hearn and Dr. Minassian review the causes, the diagnosis, and the treatments of PCOS in an easy to read, personal, and engaging manner. The personal anecdotes bring home the pain and confusion that PCOS can create in women's lives, and the need to better understand what we know, and what we do not know, about this very common disorder.

Patients with PCOS are their own best advocates, along with many physicians and nurses who are dedicated to improving the knowledge and care of these patients.

I am sure you will enjoy reading this entertaining guide to PCOS as much as I did.

Ricardo Azziz, MD, MPH, MBA

The Helping Hand Chair in Obstetrics and Gynecology
Chair, Dept. of Obstetrics and Gynecology, and
Director, Center for Androgen Related Disorders
Cedars-Sinai Medical Center

Professor and Vice-Chair,
Dept. of Obstetrics and Gynecology, and
Professor, Dept. of Medicine
The David Geffen School of Medicine at UCLA

Contents

Introduction

"I became frustrated by the lack of recognition
and understanding there is about PCOS in
the community. How many times have I told
people I have PCOS, only to have them laugh
in my face, telling me I was only making
excuses for being fat or others simply giving
me a blank stare?!"

—Jill

Hello and welcome to *Pocket PCOS*.

Since you are reading this book, you most likely have
PCOS, or know someone who does. If you are the former,
know that you're among friends who care about you. If you are
the latter, we congratulate you for taking the time and effort to
learn about this disease.

PCOS stands for Polycystic Ovary Syndrome. PCOS is
a syndrome in which the ovaries make excessive amounts of
androgen, frequently resulting in irregular periods, excessive
hair growth and infertility. PCOS is also most often, but not
always, associated with insulin resistance and obesity which
leads to increased risks for Type 2 Diabetes and coronary
artery disease.

The Prevalence of PCOS

We said you aren't alone if you suffer from PCOS but how common is the disease? The answer may depend on many factors, including how it's diagnosed or who is being diagnosed.

If ultrasound is the only method used then more than 20 percent of women in the United States have Polycystic Ovary Syndrome. If only irregular periods are used, then about 10 percent have PCOS.

It should be noted that if ultrasound alone is used, it will most assuredly give the doctor a false positive PCOS result, because some patients have the ultrasound findings but actually do not have the syndrome. So while this method is available, it is highly unreliable.

Ethnicity plays a major role as well: Caucasians and African-American women have a 4 percent incidence if PCOS, but 9 percent of Greek women suffer from it; and some research indicates that certain Latino groups have an even higher incidence. Some Native American groups have a more-than-20 percent incidence.

These statistics lead many researchers to suggest that PCOS may be an inherited problem. Insulin resistance, a major factor in dealing with PCOS, appears to be inherited too.

To translate percentages into actual numbers of people, let's use a figure of 10 percent. According to the United States Census, in 2006 there were 105,612,239 women between the ages of 15 and 69 living in America.[1] Using the figure of ten percent, there are an estimated 10.5 million (10,561,224) women in America suffering from PCOS.

Worldwide, the numbers are astronomical. In 2007 there were 2,184,262,520 women in the world between the ages of 15 and 69. If this 10 percent figure holds true worldwide, then we are looking at 21,842,625 women with PCOS in the world.[2]

So, no, you aren't alone!

For the PCOS Patient

This book is not a comprehensive guide to PCOS, but it is designed to be an excellent starting place for both the PCOS patient, and for her family and friends.

We have many goals for this book. First of all, we want to help you gain a better understanding what PCOS is and how you may be affected.

Secondly, as was said earlier, we want you to know that you are not alone. Yes, having PCOS can be scary. Yes, having PCOS can at times crush your heart (along with a dream or two). But in whatever trials and troubles PCOS takes you through, remember that you are not alone. We trust this will be evident through the many personal testimonies that are in this book.

A third goal is to help you more effectively explain PCOS to others. If you are a PCOS patient, then you know that the disease can affect very personal parts of your body and your life. This can make it difficult or embarrassing for you to talk openly about PCOS with your family and friends. That's perfectly understandable. As a starting point for explaining what PCOS is and what it means, you can give someone this book.

For Those Who Know a PCOS Patient

If you are in the group of people who knows someone who has PCOS, this book is designed to give you a better understanding of the disease. While the content and tone of the book are directed to the patient, please do not let this deter you. Reading this book will give you a much better understanding of your loved one and what she is going through. You will be given a view into the lives of several women who have PCOS. You will soon find out that this is not a "regular" disease. Women who have PCOS can feel very alone and self-conscious. They need family members, relatives and friends who will come alongside to help and support them; even defend them at times.

The Voices of PCOS

Inside these pages you will meet Amy, Rachel, Cheryl, Jill, Ruth, Jennifer and Becky. You will read in their own words what it is like for them to live with this disease.

(All the stories in this book are taken from actual women who have PCOS. Their names have been changed to protect their privacy. Only Amy's stories are adapted from various discussions that one of the authors has had with a woman who has PCOS. While some fiction has been added, Amy's stories are nonetheless accurate when describing her feelings and pain).

The stories included could be multiplied many times over. Their testimonies are just a few examples of real women who are living day in and day out with the very same disease that you have—Polycystic Ovary Syndrome.

There is strength, encouragement, and help in numbers. You are not alone. You can make it.

1. VOICES

Amy: My House Is My Prison

Amy: I can't go out. Today would be such a nice day to go to the store. I would love to get a new dress. Maybe grab a quick cup of coffee along the way, but I can't go out. Not looking like this. No way.

Jane called earlier and asked if I would like to go to a movie later tonight. How can I get myself ready in time? I would love to go—that obviously isn't the issue—but how can I make myself look halfway presentable and still make it by 6? I don't have enough time to tweeze the hairs on my cheeks and chin, and I don't want to shave. I'll just call her back and tell her I can't make it. I'll have to make something up. I hate to lie—maybe there is something I can think of and wedge into the truth?

Why does this happen to me?

Everyone thinks that I'm shy or antisocial. Actually the opposite is true! I would love to go out—shopping, movies, coffee, a walk in the park, you name it—but that isn't the life for me. My home is the only place where it is safe for me to be, where no one can see me. My house is my prison.

Why must I live like this? Living? This isn't living. How long will this last?

2. WHAT IS PCOS?

A Concise Overview of the Disease with Answers to Common Questions

First, let's start with a brief history of PCOS followed by a look at the major signs and symptoms of the disease.

Mid-1800s: French physician reported the appearance of polycystic ovaries.

1935: Two gynecologists from Chicago, Stein and Leventhal, described the symptoms of PCOS (immediately named the Stein-Leventhal Syndrome). Patients were for the most part overweight, infertile, hirsute (abnormal hair growth on the face or other parts of the body) and had a lack of menstruation (periods).

1935-2003: Many, if not most, physicians think of PCOS in the above terms.

2003: At an international conference of fertility specialists in Rotterdam, Netherlands, a new definition was agreed upon by many specialists. This Rotterdam Criteria stipulated that the following be excluded from a definition of PCOS: hormonal diseases of congenital adrenal hyperplasia (an inherited enzyme disorder), elevated prolactin, thyroid disease and Cushing's Syndrome. Then, to be diagnosed with PCOS, a patient must have two of the following three symptoms:

1. Irregular periods.

2. Elevated androgens (male hormone) either seen on the skin as acne, hirsutism (pronounced, "HIR-suit-ism"), or in actual blood tests.

3. Ultrasound findings of polycystic ovaries.

This means that you can have PCOS even if you menstruate regularly—if polycystic ovaries are seen on an ultrasound test. The Rotterdam Criteria are controversial and you may find some physicians that disagree with them.

Frequently Asked Questions

Q. What are some of the signs and symptoms of PCOS?
A. Here is a list of the most-often seen symptoms. You may be diagnosed with PCOS with just one of these symptoms. The following percentages reflect the number of women with PCOS who have the particular symptom:

1. Hirsutism (90%)

2. Menstrual irregularities/irregular periods (90%)

3. Infertility (75%)

4. Excessive weight (50%)

5. Insulin resistance (33% or more)

Q. What causes PCOS?

A. The most common opinion today among researchers is that PCOS is a syndrome with more than one cause. Two have been most often proposed:

1. Insulin resistance.

2. Some type of abnormality in the way the ovary produces hormones (androgens- a male hormone and estrogens- a female hormone).

Insulin resistance is strongly linked to PCOS. This condition occurs when the cells of your body cannot process insulin efficiently and find it hard to keep the blood sugar at a normal level. You may also be suffering from excessive weight which further aggravates the insulin resistance. In turn your body will compensate by making more insulin. This excessive insulin stimulates the ovary to make androgens and the vicious cycle is set into motion. Additionally, it may be difficult for you to lose weight when your insulin levels are elevated, further compounding the problem.

As for the second cause, some researchers have proposed that a gene defect may force the ovary into making excessive androgens. Either way, your androgens will cause follicles that are trying to mature and ovulate to stop in mid growth. The partially grown follicles collect in your ovary (making it appear polycystic) and eventually degenerate. The androgens may also cause you to have excessive hair and/or acne.

One area that is much less studied, but may be important, is the effect of stress on patients with PCOS. There have been some older and more recent reports that PCOS patients score higher on anxiety or other psychological testing. Therefore, adding stress reduction techniques looks promising to help you manage and reduce your symptoms.

Q. I may have PCOS, but I'm not sure. How can I get tested for PCOS?

A. The following is a list of several tests that your doctor can run to see if you have PCOS:

1. *Thorough physical and pelvic examination:* Checking for excess hair growth, acne, a brownish, raised skin discoloration in the body folds, and "skin tags" over the skin.

2. *Endometrial biopsy:* Ask for this test if you have a history of irregular bleeding (irregular periods) or no periods.

3. *Weight check:* "Waist-hip" ratio and "body-mass index" (BMI) to evaluate excessive weight.

4. *Blood tests:* Used to check androgen levels (testosterone, DHEA-sulfate, 17-hydroxyprogesterone, androstenedione and free testosterone, for example). Many women have increased LH (luteinizing hormone) levels compared to FSH (follicle-stimulating hormone), resulting in an elevated LH to FSH ratio.

5. *Vaginal ultrasound:* An increasingly popular test. If your ovaries are polycystic, they will be seen to be a bit enlarged and with collections of small follicle cysts lining the outer edge, just under the surface. This finding is called the "pearl necklace," "string of pearls," or "necklace" sign.

6. *Test for insulin resistance:* This is a controversial but popular test. It is the fasting glucose:insulin ratio. This test is drawn after you fast overnight and checks the baseline levels of your blood sugar and insulin. If you have a ratio less than 4.5,

that is a good indicator of insulin resistance. However, this test seems to be only 85 percent effective. Some doctors may choose to extend the test into a two-hour glucose tolerance test (GTT) with insulin levels. This test "stresses the system" to uncover the diagnosis. A fasting lipid profile (cholesterol, LDL, HDL, triglycerides) may be drawn also.

After it has been confirmed by your doctor that you have PCOS, then your next step is to receive counseling as to the risks and different treatment choices available to you. We will look at some of the main options throughout this book. Even if you have only recently been diagnosed with PCOS, do not despair! There is hope for you and all who suffer under this disease.

Q. Can I just ignore my PCOS, and hope nothing bad will happen to me?

A. This is not a recommended course for you to take. PCOS carries with it both short- and long-term risks.

Rachel says, "PCOS was a big deal—and was causing many of my health problems. PCOS steals away the control over your own body. It drives you to obsess about it. It seems you are always at its mercy, destined to struggle against the normal tides."

Alexandra says, "I was having serious mood swings; they were awful. If you were talking to me one minute, the next I could be throwing a cup your way. My husband was beside himself; I was a Jekyll and Hyde. I was bursting into tears at any time and then would just want to be left alone."

In one 9 year period, Alexandra had three breakdowns. She had been off work for six months out of one year, and four months out of another year.

Alexandra even came up with a "mood meter" so her husband would know instantly how she was feeling. Her grades were A, B or C.

(A) *Absolutely devastated.* Not focusing on anything but wanting a baby. Dreading going out and seeing children. Not being able to cope with day-to-day life. Everything is unbearable, including simple tasks like taking a shower.

(B) *Being brave.* Trying to remain positive and hope for the best. Take a 'Let's see what happens' attitude.

(C) *Calm and really considering the question*—'Did I want a child or did I just want to overcome PCOS?' Trying and convince herself that her life was all right and to be grateful for the things she had, a good marriage for example.

"As you can see, to say I cope well with this illness is a lie! I suffer with depression, anxiety, stress, all the side effects of PCOS—I've got them all—acne, irregular periods, facial hair, skin tags, brown patches, insulin problems, joint aches, water retention, hair thinning, I dare not go on. This illness is the hardest thing I have had to accept in my life."

In the short term, PCOS can cause infertility and uncontrolled or irregular vaginal bleeding (dysfunctional uterine bleeding) with the possibility of anemia.

If you suffer from insulin resistance, you will have a much higher risk of Type 2 (adult type) diabetes later in life. You also have a higher risk for dyslipidemias: high blood levels of cholesterol or other lipid substances. High blood pressure is more common too. For this reason, most PCOS researchers feel that there is a higher rate of heart disease and atherosclerosis if you have PCOS.

Cancer of the endometrium is a long-term risk that has been known for decades. As a woman with PCOS, your body does not make enough estrogen to grow your endometrium (much of it from your own body fat), and without regular shedding of the lining, the endometrium can grow uncontrollably. Without ovulation there is no progesterone (which is the hormone of ovulation) to oppose this effect of the estrogen. After many years this "unopposed estrogen" may lead to a precancerous condition called hyperplasia, which may eventually lead you to have cancer.

One new area of research has looked at the risks for pregnancy complications in women with PCOS once they conceive. Miscarriage rates seem to be higher and may be related to the higher androgen or LH levels. Also, the risk for gestational diabetes can run up to 30 percent if you have PCOS.

While it is never pleasant to deal with health problems, action is the best policy to follow.

3. VOICES

A Poem: *Hormones*

The following poem was written by a woman who has PCOS. Maybe it describes what you are going through.

HORMONES

I know I'm not going crazy

Although it seems to be

That nothing is making sense at all

I just don't feel like me

Many tears I've shed,

To friends down the phone

Crying over little things,

letting out a moan

I feel that I am useless.

Am no good to anyone

I've lost control of my emotions

And want something to be done

I've been calling out for help,

but it seems I've not been heard

Doctors send me away,

without a single word

My blood sugars are high,

as I expected them to be

but nothing could prepare me

for the truth that was meant to be.

Its hit me very hard,

like a punch and kick to the gut

Really took me by surprise

I feel like such a mutt.

Going through the change???

The doctor said to me,

as one test showed I was up and down,

The other as clear can be.

Doctors have no idea, of what I'm going through.

I spend each night crying

and trying to think things through.

I'm sick of feeling out of control,

I want to bring ME back.

I used to be soo happy,

I feel so out of whack.

I go to my hubby for support,

he just doesn't know what to do.

He suggests that I don't give up work

But wants me happy too.

I really don't know what to do,

my head is in a mess.

Blurting out and crying,

I have been trying to confess.

Not that I have things to hide,

I'm a fairly open chick.

But when I cant handle things anymore,

I need a little kick.

I know that I'm not crazy,

my emotions are everywhere

I've leant on my friends & family,

for support and they have been there.

—February 2, 2004

4. VOICES

Amy: Why Can't I Have Kids?

Amy: As a young woman with PCOS, I don't have any kids. The doctors have assured me that unless I take infertility medicine, there would be no way that I would be able to have kids. Their diagnosis was in essence, "Don't even think about it."

I've always wanted to have kids; at least one child. Yet I don't like the idea of taking infertility medicine to become pregnant. I mean, that's fine for some women—I'm not judging them— but for me, I've never been comfortable with going that route. I've heard of women who couldn't conceive naturally, took infertility medicine, then ended up being pregnant with three or more kids at once! Yiiiipes!

Adoption is another option, but I've always wanted to give birth to my own baby. Not to frown on those who chose to adopt, it's a wonderful and beautiful act of love. For now, though, it's not something that my husband and I are considering.

I feel empty and not quite right, knowing that I will never be able to have a baby naturally. I feel less than whole. I am less than a full woman. I see a woman with her baby in the stroller. My heart sinks and the tears start to rise.

Why can't I be that woman? Why can't that be my baby in the stroller?

5. INFERTILITY

Part 1

PCOS is a significant cause of infertility. In fact, it is the number one cause of infertility in women in the United States.

PCOS increases androgen levels in the ovary, which causes a lack of ovulation, or irregular ovulation. The unnatural level of androgen interferes with the normal growth of follicles, which are cysts carrying eggs (ova) in the ovary. You are born with millions of ova which develop into follicles during normal cycles. One of these follicles eventually releases the egg (ovulation) creating fertility. PCOS reduces your odds of becoming pregnant by reducing the number of ovulation cycles per year.

The syndrome can also cause minor ovulation defects; even cycles that appear ovulatory could be less than ideal for fertility if you are not under treatment.

PERSONAL EXPERIENCES

To have a doctor tell you that you can not conceive can be heart-crushing. A hope that's been dreamed about since childhood has been dashed to the ground.

Let's read how some women struggle with infertility. Later in the book we will see the results at their attempts to become pregnant.

After marrying, Rachel decided to stop birth control. She says that she and her husband "were not actively trying to conceive but agreed that we did not want to prevent conception." Six years passed, and the situation became painful:

> Our families were starting to ask when we were going to have children — almost demanding that we give them a date. We started out explaining details, I have PCOS, this is what PCOS means there will have to be costly fertility treatments and so on. I didn't feel complete; I felt like a freak and a failure as a woman. Eventually it was just easier to tell people I couldn't conceive. Being overweight and carrying most of the bulge in my stomach area, it was common at reunions to be asked when I was due. I was being stabbed with a double edge sword.

Ruth says that her husband and she "have tried unsuccessfully for fourteen years to conceive and had experienced four miscarriages and three failed IVF [in vitro fertilization—*ed*.] attempts. I had been on Clomid and Metformin and also underwent infertility operations such as ovarian drilling, a histogram and laparoscopy. You name it, we did it."

Becky says she did not understand what PCOS was, and was beginning to think that she was never going to have children. After seeing a new doctor, she writes:

> I was immediately started on Glucophage, and
> started charting my temperature to see if I was
> ovulating. Several months had passed with no
> ovulation. I was so upset, I thought that I was
> being punished, and that God would never
> give me a child. It seemed everyone around
> me was getting pregnant. I was so upset,
> even mad at them. I didn't understand how
> two married people who loved each other so
> much could not get pregnant when there are
> fourteen-year-olds and drug addicts getting
> pregnant.

After this, Becky tried Prometrium and Clomid but nothing happened. Month after month Becky tried this treatment without success for three years.

Alexandra started IVF procedures in 1997. She says of the experience,

It was awful. The drugs they gave me made me ill and I was vomiting all the time. Phil, my husband, was really good and did the injections. Unfortunately, my body did not respond well enough to the drugs; hardly any follicles had grown and the lining on my womb was not thick enough, so the treatment was suspended. I was devastated. I don't even remember coming home from the hospital. I was unbearable to live with; I was so depressed and suffered a nervous breakdown.

Alexandra's sister had two children, which was difficult for Alexandra to take.

> Don't get me wrong, I love my sister to bits,
> but I felt so jealous and green with envy that
> she had kids and I had none. My sister was so
> considerate when she was carrying her child,
> but I was devastated. I was the eldest and yet
> I wanted to be the first to produce the first
> grandchild. In all of her pregnancies not once
> did she make me feel uncomfortable or hurt
> and I adore and love her for that so much.

Nevertheless, Alexandra started to distant herself from others who were pregnant and had lost many friends who started a family. She wanted to give her husband children. To face such obstacles was very difficult for her. She says,

> I am a very maternal person and have always
> been so successful in everything else I have
> done, but putting a child on this earth seemed
> out of my control. This always broke my
> heart because I always felt I was born to be a
> mother. I know others feel the same way and
> you are not alone!

Jennifer also had to deal with the difficulty of hearing that she would never naturally have kids, and at a young age. She writes,

> It was around the 8th grade, I was visiting one of my doctors. I don't remember what kind of doctor he was, only that I didn't really care for him. I remember him telling me very insensitively that I would *never* have children.
>
> Imagine you're a preteen girl, who's probably just started thinking about her future life. You'll go to college, get a job, get married, have a family, and live happily ever after, the end. To hear that I would never have kids was quite heartbreaking, because I'd always work with children—from being a teacher's aide to all the babysitting, to working in a daycare—and I was going to be a grade school teacher when I grew up! I most certainly wanted to bring my own children into my life, but he said I wouldn't!
>
> I was heartbroken for several years, until I finally decided that I *will* have children if I really want to. Fortunately I now see a doctor who's a bit more realistic; he told me that it may be difficult to conceive on my own, but not impossible, because he certainly can't see the future, and stranger things have happened.

As you can see and perhaps personally know yourself, it can be very disheartening to hear that you will never have children. Yet there are options. We've read of women who have tried different infertility treatments with the hopes that one will work and enable them to conceive. Others have also looked into adoption as a way to have children. We will read what happens with each of these women later in the book.

REASONS FOR HOPE

If you want to become pregnant, options are available. Your treatment plan should be customized to your individual situation. The recent explosion of research in PCOS and its connection with insulin resistance has added more and better treatment options for patients. Here is a summary:

1. *Clomiphene citrate* (trade names, "Clomid" or "Serophene"), which is usually prescribed with Metformin (an insulin sensitizer). Ovulation rates are up to 90 percent and average pregnancy rates of 50 percent have been seen.

2. *Taking Metformin* alone. While this is an option, testing shows that using Metformin alone for fertility treatments is not as effective as combining it with Clomiphene.

3. *Injectable gonadotropins.* Generally used in cases of failure to ovulate with Clomiphene. These medications include the hormones FSH (trade names Follistim, Bravelle, Gonal-F) or a combination of FSH and LH (trade name Menopur or Repronex). Ovulation rates for injectable gonadotropins are over 90 percent and pregnancy rates are approximately 50 percent.

4. *Ovarian drilling.* Many women who undergo this procedure will eventually return to having irregular periods.

5. *Diet modification and exercise.* An example would be a reduced carbohydrate diet, and regular, structured exercise.

Of course, you should consider looking at other reasons for infertility before committing to fertility treatments for PCOS.

A semen analysis (sperm count) is recommended to see if the problem is with the male. For women, a common procedure is to have the fallopian tubes checked with a rapid x-ray screening test called an HSG (hysterosalpingogram), in which dye is injected into the uterus and seen to flow out of the tubes on a monitor screen. Also, a laparoscopy can be performed, in which a small incision is made in the umbilicus and a scope with a video connection is inserted to further evaluate the inside of the pelvis. This is normally a short, same-day surgical procedure performed under general anesthesia.

6. VOICES

Jennifer: I Can't Lose Weight

Jennifer: "I was a soccer referee starting around age thirteen, I think, and I became a coach at age fifteen. Yet I was still unable to lose any weight, even though I was at soccer practice four days a week; two as coach and two as a player.

I have always been a chubby girl, even when I was very physically active. I started taking dance lessons at age four, and quit at age ten to start playing soccer. I played indoor and outdoor soccer until I was sixteen or seventeen. I was a soccer referee starting around age thirteen, I think, and I became a coach at age fifteen. Yet I was still unable to lose any weight, even though I was at soccer practice four days a week; two as coach and two as a player. I was out on the fields all day on Saturday too, but still…

Jennifer recalls that she was teased in high school because of her weight. People would say, "Mooo!" when she walked by or would pretend an earthquake struck as she sat down.

PCOS has affected every aspect of my life—in bad ways, and in good ways. For a very long time, I was very self-conscious of my looks, because I wasn't some stick-thin model who starved herself to death to conform to society's mold of being beautiful. It took me a very long time to get over that feeling.

I had a good number of friends who liked to tell me in high school how fat they were, and how much weight they needed to lose, to be pretty. These girls were smaller than me; a great deal smaller. They took diet pills, starved themselves, whatever, to achieve the look they thought they needed to have. When I reminded them that they were so much smaller than I was, and that if they thought themselves fat, how must the see me—I was always told that I wasn't fat, I was just fine.

Nobody ever understood how much that hurt me. Sure, in their eyes nothing was wrong with me, but how did they affect me?

7. WEIGHT GAIN

Being overweight can be very difficult for anyone, but perhaps most especially for a teenager or young woman. This can be especially true when you know that your weight gain is not because of overeating. It can also be maddening to lose weight, only to gain it back again.

It's easy to say that people who are overweight are so because they overeat and are lazy. This is not always true. There are often many other factors. PCOS, for example, can make it very hard, if not impossible, for women to lose weight. This is not a cop-out, but a medical fact.

Perhaps the woman in your office or your next door neighbor is overweight. Maybe she has PCOS and despite keeping a rigid diet and exercising, she just can't keep the pounds off. She is doing the best she can to lose weight, but is being held back by the disease.

Since PCOS symptoms frequently are first noticed after large weight gains, many doctors believe that weight gain will actually trigger the syndrome.

As we said at the beginning of the book, insulin resistance is the key to understanding the problem of weight gain. It is now well known that most women with PCOS, if not the vast majority, are insulin resistant, and many are obese. The area of insulin resistance is where you should focus your attention if obesity is one of your symptoms.

PERSONAL EXPERIENCES

Here's what Rachel says:

> I have always been overweight as are most of the members of my family; male and female. I tried diets throughout my teen years based on whatever my mother was currently trying and had moderate success. Yet after stopping the strict regimen, the weight would return.
>
> I also developed asthma after getting pneumonia following a tonsillectomy. This made exercising difficult until I was able to get it under control. I lost the most weight during my first year in college. I stopped eating almost completely and exercised daily by walking at the track or using the weight room. I was following an anorexic style but still did not drop to even an ideal weight.
>
> I remember being so excited that I could squeeze into a pair of size 12's that summer. Until that point I had joked that my age was always my jeans' size. That has remained true from age 6 to 30 with this one exception."

Ruth writes,

My weight went out of control and seemed to get in the way of everything. So I went to a seminar about PCOS and a lecture took place about how our metabolism is affected by PCOS and we need to treat it.

So I went on a hunt for someone who knew about metabolic diets, et cetera. I had tried everything, Weight Watchers, Slimmer's World, you name it, and I had done it. Anyway I discovered an organization called Vitaline and went and did their plan for a week and lost seven pounds. Within six weeks I had lost over thirty-eight pounds and felt great."

REASONS FOR HOPE

If you have PCOS and want to lose weight, then insulin resistance must be reduced. The good news is that it is possible to "turn back time" and reverse the process. There are medications, including those used to combat Type 2 diabetes, that are very helpful in reducing insulin resistance. The most commonly prescribed medication is Metformin (with the brand names off Glucophage or Fortamet).

Glucophage is the most studied and most prescribed. It is at least 75 percent effective in recent studies. Many patients will report some weight loss initially on this drug.

Side effects, especially with Metformin, can occur, and therefore you must always check with your doctor to see if you are at risk for one or more of these effects. Pioglitazone (Actos) and Rosiglitazone (Avandia) are less studied but can provide an alternative to Metformin.

Insulin sensitizers (like Metformin) can be given to allow for regular periods, help in weight loss and prevent the long-term effects of PCOS. The sensitizers will let ovulation occur, so if you are sexually active, you must use care to avoid unwanted pregnancies. In fact, some specialists are using oral contraceptives and sensitizers together to prevent this for such patients.

In addition to medication, lifestyle modification is crucial. The categories of diets most often recommended include low carbohydrate plans and calorie restriction plans. Healthy, consistent weight loss combines using a medicine like Metformin with diet modification and exercise.

Many weight loss franchises now offer specific plans for PCOS. Whether you use a book or class, make sure that the resource uses a plan that specifically targets PCOS. Ask your doctor and others who have PCOS as to their current treatment plans.

Exercise is an extremely important modification. Regular aerobic exercise, increasing the heart rate and achieving endurance, is essential for you to achieve consistent and successful weight loss.

Finding enjoyable, long-term ways to reduce stress is advisable as well

Using all four interventions—medicine, exercise, diet, stress reduction—is the key to success for many overweight PCOS patients.

For women with severe obesity, gastric bypass surgery may be recommended as a treatment option. New techniques like laparoscopic gastric bypass surgery have reduced the complication rates from the procedure. Nevertheless it's a decision you must thoroughly explore with your physician.

USEFUL WEBSITES

Methods for losing weight:
The Atkins diet- http://atkins.com
Jenny Craig, Inc.- http://www.jennycraig.com
Slim-Fast- http://www.slim-fast.com
The South Beach Diet- http://www.southbeachdiet.com/
    index3.asp
Sugar Busters- http://www.sugarbusters.com
Vitaline- http://www.vitaline-slimming.com
Weight Watchers- http://www.weightwatchers.com
A natural approach- http://www.weightlossforall.com

Articles on how to lose weight, especially geared for women with PCOS can be found at:
http://www.soulcysters.com/weight_loss.html
http://www.weightloss.about.com/od/morediet1/a/
    aa051005a.htm.

RECOMMENDED BOOKS

Arthur Agatston, *The South Beach Diet: The Delicious, Doctor-Designed, Foolproof Plan for Fast and Healthy Weight Loss* (St. Martin's Griffin, 2005).

Arthur Agatston, *The South Beach Diet Dining Guide: Your Reference Guide to Restaurants Across America* (Rodale, 2005).

Arthur Agatston, *The South Beach Diet Quick and Easy Cookbook: 200 Delicious Recipes Ready in 30 Minutes or Less* (Rodale, 2005).

8. VOICES

Amy: Too Much Hair

Amy: I feel cursed. Maybe God is punishing me for something. What did I do to deserve this disease? I feel so alone. Surely no one is suffering like I am. I look around at everyone—laughing, going here and there, no problems at all. Not like me. Regular women get up, maybe do a quick five to ten minutes of make-up, comb their hair, and off they go. But not me.

I would love to be able to get up and go after just ten minutes of getting ready. Ten minutes! I have to set the alarm for 5:00 a.m., even though my meeting doesn't start until nine. If I was normal I could sleep until eight. I can't believe I have to spend a whole three hours in front of the mirror. Plucking and tweezing. Plucking and tweezing. What a way to start the day.

My thumb hurts and aches. I can barely hold the tweezers any longer and I'm still not finished; I still have more to go. I should just grow a beard and become a man! Why not? The way people look and stare at me—some even ask me what's wrong with my face.

I can't win. I go out either with a bit of growth, which is visible, or I go out with red marks from tweezing, which are visible.

It's not fair. Why me? Why, God? Some days it's just not worth it. I refuse to do it and stay inside. If only the growth was limited to my arms and legs, then I could cover up with clothing and not have to worry about shaving or tweezing. Sure, I would get hot at times, but it's so much quicker and easier than worrying about my face.

Maybe I could try plastic surgery. I could get new skin put on the old and then the hair wouldn't grow anymore. I hear that there are women with PCOS who are dealing with hair loss! How ironic.

9. HAIR GROWTH

As we have already mentioned, excessive hair growth (hirsutism) is another possible and common symptom of PCOS. As you may well know, when this growth is on your face and neck, it can feel absolutely horrifying.

Do you spend hours upon hours plucking and tweezing? Have you spent many a dollar on electrolysis or laser treatment? You're not alone.

PERSONAL EXPERIENCES

Here's what Rachel says:

> I had hair everywhere. Two incidents stand out vividly in my mind.
>
> I was sitting on the curb and my mother approached and told me that with the way the sun was hitting me my dad had noticed how much facial hair I had, and told her to get me to do something about it. That is horrifying to a sixteen-year-old.
>
> In college a group of girls, including my roommate, commented on the amount

of forearm hair a couple of us had, saying
how gross it was. There were jokes about
bears, gorillas and other furry creatures that
followed.

When waxing and chemical removers had
no effect other than to leave me with burns for
several days, I resorted to shaving my face and
arms everyday. My hair has become darker
over the years so even with this daily shaving
I often appear to have stubble or irritated
bumps.

One day a young girl I was mentoring
reached up to touch my face one day and
snatched her hand back in shock when she felt
the shaved area. I moisturize but it will never
be smooth and beautiful.

Jennifer says she remembers "growing the hair I shouldn't
have":

It was seventh grade and I had just switched
from a Catholic school to the local public
junior high. Some of the boys who sat near
me in my firs-hour English class thought it
was quite amusing to tell me that I needed to
shave, or that I had more facial hair than their
older brother or father or whomever they felt
like comparing me to that day. Yeah, I would
usually tell them to come back when they'd
successfully grown a brain, but their taunts
still hurt.

In the eighth grade, a really rotten boy somehow got hold of my yearbook and drew a beard and mustache on my picture. My mom complained to my principal, but all he really said was "boys will be boys" and left him unpunished. Oh, he did offer to trade books with me, but mine was already signed by all my friends and as much as I hated that picture, I didn't want to lose the good memories. So somewhere among my things is my eighth-grade yearbook picture, complete with hand-drawn graffiti. I'm sure I'll jump at the chance to show that to my children.

Alexandra comments,

I was shaving my face nearly every day, I was trying to hide it and having to use a razor everyday. I have stubble just like a man and now we have his and her shavers.

On the other side, you may suffer from hair loss. Incredible isn't it? You have either too much hair or too little. What a cruel disease indeed, it is a disease that mocks you. Weight gain, infertility, acne, hair loss or growth- it hits you in some of the major areas where it means to be a woman.

REASONS FOR HOPE

If you suffer from hirsutism, take heart that it can be very well suppressed with oral contraceptives together with the drug Spironolactone, which lowers androgens. Vaniqa, a prescription cream, looks somewhat effective as well.

Many women have found one or a combination of the following to help them control hirsutism:

1. *Shaving*

2. *Waxing*

3. *Tweezing*

4. *Electrolysis*

5. *Laser treatment.* Laser hair removal is an excellent option, though it can be quite expensive and rarely permanent if you have PCOS.

6. *Eflornithine* (Vaniqa). This is a topical cream that is available only by prescription. Eflornithine helps some women reduce the rate of facial hair growth. It is applied twice a day to the face, on the areas of excess hair growth. Results with Eflornithine are mixed; some patients note good results while others may not.

7. *Insulin sensitizers*: Metformin (Glucophage, Fortamet), Pioglitazone (Actos), Avandia (Rosiglitazone). These medications help reduce insulin resistance and as a result lower androgen levels coming from the ovaries. This means that they can help reduce hirsutism as well as regulate periods and help you to lose weight. Diet modification and regular exercise are needed to get the greatest benefit from these medications (see Chapter 6). [6]

8. *Cyproterone*. This is an anti-androgen medication. It reduces androgen levels and in turn, hirsutism.

9. *Spironolactone* (Aldactone). This has been used for many years as a very effective medication to control hirsutism in PCOS patients, and is actually a diuretic used to treat hypertension. It works best when used in conjunction with oral contraceptives. Spironolactone can also be used together with Metformin for a better overall effect. Because it lowers androgens, this medication can allow more regular periods to occur.

10. *Flutamide and Finasteride*. These are also anti-androgen medications. They have similar effects to Spironolactone and Cyproterone for hirsutism and their use seems to be relatively free of side effects. They are not routinely prescribed for PCOS patients; however when they are, they should be used in conjunction with a method of contraception. Like spironolactone and flutamide they actually work better with oral contraceptives.

11. *Birth control pill* (Oral contraceptives). Production of androgens by the ovaries can be suppressed with oral contraceptives. This can lead to lower levels of free testosterone. Since the therapy requires at least six months for a visible effect, shaving, waxing, and so on, can be used in the meantime. In particular, Diane-35 (Cyproterone) and Estelle-35 have been specifically made to work against male hormones. It works best when used with Spironolactone. Check with your doctor to see which kind of pill is best for you.

12. *Natural remedies*. Quite a number of vitamins and minerals have been claimed helpful for normalizing insulin

and androgens, or reducing the effects of testosterone. They include chromium picolinate (reduces insulin resistance), cinnamon extract, vitamin E, magnesium, zinc, copper and vitamin B6, to name a few. It remains to be seen if there is any scientific proof to their claims.

There are herbal medicines that may work like anti-androgen drugs by inhibiting the enzyme that converts testosterone into the much more potent DHT (dihydrotestosterone). DHT is the hormone in your skin that stimulates hirsutism. Serenoa repens (saw palmetto), pygeum africans (15) and urtica dioica (stinging nettles) all inhibit the action of testosterone. There have been many studies of men with testosterone disorders that demonstrate the effectiveness and safety of these herbs. There aren't any studies of hirsute PCOS women as yet, so the effectiveness of these treatments has not been established. Nonetheless, it may be worth it for you to talk to your doctor about such remedies.

USEFUL WEBSITES

Advanced Fertility Center of Chicago- http://www.advancedfertility.com

The American Electrology Association- http://www.electrology.com

HairFacts, an independent website dedicated to looking at how to control hair growth- http://www.hairfacts.com

Vaniqa- http://www.vaniqa.com

Polycystic Ovarian Syndrome Association-

http://www.pcosupport.org/news/PCOSBulletin-June2005.
pdf. (PCOS Bulletin. Volume 8, issue 1, June, 2005.
Page 5 from this bulletin gives a nice, concise look at the
differences in the major hair removal methods.)

U.S. Food and Drug Administration website which looks at
laser treatment- http://www.fda.gov/cdrh/consumer/
laserfacts.html

10. VOICES

Becky: Pregnant!

Becky:

I had blood drawn on a Friday. Monday I called to see if they had the results. The nurse said the lab was backed up and they would call me. I thought, 'Okay no problem.' The next Friday morning I called back and the nurse was busy, so I left a message. I was so frustrated, I thought I was going to have to wait and agonize over the weekend. At 4:30 that day I got a call from the nurse....I was pregnant!! I couldn't believe it!

At the first sonogram I found out that I was having twins! I had never known such happiness than to see those two tiny dots on the screen. The boys were born three months early and weighed 2 lb. 8 oz, and 2 lb. 7 oz. After staying in the ICU for six weeks they were able to come home.

11. INFERTILITY

Part 2

In chapter 5 we heard about struggles our PCOS women faced to become pregnant. Now let's check in and see how these ladies are doing.

Amy shares her success story.

> I had stopped planning or thinking about conceiving and giving birth. After all, two doctors on two different occasions told me that I had a 0 percent chance of conceiving without the use of infertility drugs. Even though we are Christians, we weren't even praying to God to help us to conceive. Nonetheless, God blessed us with a healthy baby girl who weighed 8 pounds, 7 ounces. This was truly a medical miracle.

Ruth reports that she and her husband decided to pursue adoption, "We were thankfully matched with a beautiful little girl called Lynn who we adored the first day we met her. The day we collected her to take her home for good, I received a phone call to say I needed to contact my consultant. He needed to prescribe something for me to achieve a period and instructed me as he normally did to do a pregnancy test before he could prescribe. We did and to our amazement it was positive. Six and a half months later Jill arrived; three weeks early. We became parents within six months to two beautiful little girls we adore."

Alexandra has a similar story.

We adopted our little girl. Yes, we were accepted, and [I found] out I was pregnant the same day we collected my little girl. [It] was so overwhelming. I cannot put into words how I felt that day. Susan, my miracle, was born. I sobbed for weeks and even now cannot believe I am the proud mommy of two beautiful daughters. I had the luck of receiving two babies in six months and it has been very hard to adapt, but I would not swap it for the world. I cannot believe that after all this time of trying it has happened to us. I still have to pinch myself.

Sadly, not all of our PCOS women have success stories to share. Listen to Rachel.

In March of 2005, the same day as our talk with the doctor, my husband's sister died of cancer. He lost his job and was drifting without an anchor. The more I talked of fertility the further he pulled away.
In my mind we were racing against a timeline and our chances of conceiving were getting slimmer by the minute. He felt it was

wrong to even see the specialist. I was over
300 pounds and I had to lose weight before
we would be able to conceive as it would not
be safe at this weight. I explained that we
needed to develop habits such as charting
and that we were not going to be expecting a
child right away. My husband and I stopped
spending time together. I would continue to
forward PCOS related articles to his e-mail
but we had stopped discussing options.

   He no longer lives with me. It is very
difficult at this stage to think of going through
with a divorce.

As you can see, Rachel's struggle and desire to become
pregnant must deal with the reality that her biological clock
is ticking. If she gets divorced, then she would need to find
another partner, losing even more time, and a new partner
brings no guarantees of conceiving.

   Still, there are solid reasons to hope that one day you may
give birth to your baby boy or girl.   Jennifer writes,

   Jim, our son, was born. The doctor took
him out and briefly showed his gooey, blue
face to me over the drape. [My husband]
Roger tells me that when they placed him
on the table to clean him and warm him, he
grabbed the blanket and started chewing on it.
That's something he did pretty frequently, and
something he still does. When Jim arrived,
his eyes were wide open, and he was taking

everything in. From the start, he was a nosey baby, in everyone's business. We knew right from the start he was going to be an active baby, and probably quite a handful. We were right. He was 7 pounds, 2.3 ounces, and was 20 inches long. We were overjoyed with our little one.

USEFUL WEBSITES

American Society for Reproductive Medicine website explores infertility and other topics- http://www.asrm.org

The InterNational Council on Infertility Information Dissemination, Inc.- http://www.inciid.org

The National Infertility Association- http://www.resolve.org

The Society of Reproductive Endocrinology and Infertility- http://www.socrei.org

Vitaline's PCOS website- http://www.vitaline-slimming.com/pcos

Postings, blogs and other information regarding infertility- http://www.fertilethoughts.net/ft/infertility

12. VOICES

Jennifer: I Am Not A Moron

Jennifer: While in school I remember that my parents had to fight insurance a lot to cover treatment for me. I had detached myself from this whole process because it seemed as if all the doctors thought I was a stupid moron, and never wanted to explain what was happening to me.

13. DOCTORS, GOOD AND BAD

Only recently has PCOS been recognized by doctors as a disease of its own. Still, not all doctors or OBGYNs know of PCOS or how to help you. In fact, there seems to be more doctors who do not know of PCOS than those who do.

Does your doctor know you have PCOS? Does he or she recognize PCOS and work with you on treatment options?

Some of the women in this book have run into a few doctors who do not know of PCOS. Rachel says, "I told every doctor I had of the PCOS diagnosis. None really understood it. I had assumed from my diagnosing OBGYN that it was not that big of a deal."

> One day in the hospital waiting room, I came across an article on PCOS. The article profiled three women with PCOS and told of their struggles. I was so taken aback—they looked just like me! PCOS was a big deal—and was causing many of my health problems. There was a recommended treatment called Metformin; an insulin drug. I started researching on the Internet and bringing copies into my doctor appointments.

My general practitioner read the articles but didn't see how it applied to him. He saw my condition as a fertility issue and recommended that I see the OBGYN for the prescription for Metformin. My OBGYN felt that as it was an insulin drug and blood levels would need monitoring and I needed to see my general practitioner. I was trapped in this horrible ping pong game.

My general practitioner finally agreed to check my hormone levels. All my sugar related levels were in normal range. I had already been watching what I ate as my cholesterol was high. Even though I had articles from medical journals stating that it was common for women with PCOS to have normal sugar levels and that they still experienced progress with Metformin, he refused to prescribe it. He suggested diet and exercise.

I was already doing this and not losing any weight. It took me over three months to lose fifteen pounds eating 1,500 calories a day with moderate daily exercise. I was hungry, moody and my periods had stopped again. I gave up. I didn't see the point in taking care of myself anymore. I saw it as preventing me from getting the help I needed; and that is a really messed up emotional place to be.

Becky writes of a time when she was in the hospital because one of her cysts on an ovary burst.

The hospital referred me to a doctor for a follow up, since I didn't have an OBGYN. They did a series of blood tests and confirmed that I indeed did have PCOS. That doctor didn't explain it to me or offer any medical advice. He knew that I was trying to conceive, and wouldn't even prescribe something to induce a period.

After several months of seeing him and him doing nothing for me, I started looking for a new doctor. The second doctor I saw was not what I was looking for either. I did not know much about PCOS. At this point I was beginning to get frustrated. I still did not really understand what PCOS was and was beginning to think that I was never going to have children. My search continued for a doctor that actually knew what PCOS was and that knew how to treat it.

Do any of these stories sound familiar? Has something similar happened to you?

As we have seen, PCOS is a disease with its own symptoms and plans for control. Unfortunately, there is no one cure for PCOS. We hope one day there will be. Until then, there are different treatment plans, medicines and natural remedies that you can use to manage your symptoms.

If you have or think that you may have PCOS, ask questions of your current doctor or OBGYN. If you are not satisfied with their answers, seek out a doctor who recognizes PCOS as a real disease. There are doctors who are knowledgeable and experienced in helping women with PCOS. A good start to finding a good PCOS doctor is to browse the websites listed at the end of this chapter.

In addition, talk to other teens or women via PCOS chat forums on the Internet. Remember that you are not alone; there are others who have PCOS and suffer too. A list of such chat rooms can be found in the chapter on resources. While you always want to double-check with a doctor any medical information you receive in a chat room, they can be great places to hear of different methods of treatment that work well or not so well. Reach out to others with PCOS, and you can be a source of help and encouragement to others too. The better informed you will be, the better you will be able to manage your PCOS.

It is encouraging to see that there are doctors that do see PCOS as a disease, with its own symptoms and possible means for control and management. Even if you have to drive for an hour or two, it is worth it to go to such a doctor or physician.

Jennifer writes,

> I am very fortunate that I have a wonderful endocrinologist, whom I've been seeing since high school or longer, and a great OBGYN who specializes in high-risk pregnancies, of which all of mine will be. Both doctors have been monitoring me very closely, and are

taking extra good care of me; unfortunately, many women have yet to find this luxury.

Becky says, "My search continued for a doctor who actually knew what PCOS was and knew how to treat it. With my third doctor I found a keeper! He took his time and explained PCOS to me. He was shocked that I had such bad experiences with the first two doctors."

Alexandra says, "My doctor was fantastic and will notice things, like if I have lost weight and if I have changed the color of my hair."

USEFUL WEBSITES

Cedars Sinai where Dr. Ricardo Azziz works: http://www.cedars-sinai.edu

The IVF-Fertility Program of the Women's Clinic, Ltd., Reading, PA., where Dr. Shahab S. Minassian practices: www.infertilitypa.com.

A list of doctors who are members of the Polycystic Ovarian Syndrome Association (Please keep in mind that this list is not exhaustive of all good or knowledgeable PCOS doctors) can be found at- http://www.pcosupport.org/membership/professionals.php.

The American Society for Reproductive Medicine: www.asrm.org

Androgen Excess and PCOS Society: www.androgenexcesssociety.org

INCIID: www.inciid.org

PCOSA: www.pcosupport.org

RESOLVE: The National Infertility Association: www. resolve.org

Soul Cysters: www.soulcysters.com

14. VOICES

Jennifer: Help At Last!

Jennifer: "I am also very fortunate that my husband is so supportive throughout all of this. He's gone to every one of my appointments to visit both my endocrinologist and my OBGYN. I'm glad for that, as PCOS really affects him too and the more he knows how to help me through this, the more we can help each other."

15. PCOS SUPPORT

Receiving help and standing tall with PCOS.

Your coworker, friend, spouse, daughter—any of these people could have PCOS. If you know someone who suffers from PCOS, she needs your support and understanding. If you have PCOS, you know how easy it is to feel ashamed of your body because of one or more of the symptoms PCOS can bring. Remember that you are not the disease; do not let PCOS define who you are. You are deserving of help and support.

Ruth says, "I have a very good relationship with my husband as far as communication goes. It was very hard at first but pursuing adoption helped us be more open to each other. Sometimes we held back our true emotions, hoping we would not hurt each other's feelings because infertility was such a raw subject in our marriage. I'm sure it is in other people's marriages too."

Alexandra says, "I have a fantastic husband but feel that he hides his feelings to keep from hurting me. We have been to counseling and it helped me to break down and admit that I often thought he was going to leave me. I even said to him that if we didn't have children in our life by the time I was 35, I wanted out of the marriage so he could meet someone else. Going through the adoption process brought us so much closer."

Jennifer shares her perspective stressing the importance of important education.

PCOS is not only a hereditary disease, but some statistics show that nearly 5-15 percent of the female population is affected by it. That means that there is a very good likelihood that someone you know has it. Unfortunately, she may or may not be getting treatment for it.

I know that some of the women in my family have some form of it or another, and I worry a great deal. I have seen firsthand what can happen to women and their families if this disease is left untreated and if people are left uninformed. The results can be devastating— lack of adequate treatment can ultimately lead to death by complications such as heart disease or diabetes, just to name a couple.

I am taking it upon myself to educate as many people as I possibly can, so that maybe more women will be able to get treatment without having to fight their doctors, their insurance companies and their families.

I would like people to think about how they treat others. There is a lot more to people than most of us could ever know by taking a casual glance at them. What I do want, though, is support. This is not always an easy road to travel, for my husband, myself, or anyone else in my family, but it is made easier by people who truly understand what's going on.

The diagnosis of PCOS may bring you a lot of questions, frustrations, and anxiety. Physicians are important, but they are not the only source of counseling and information available to you. You can turn to support and advocacy groups such as the Polycystic Ovarian Syndrome Association, which maintains a chapter in nearly every large city in the United States. To contact a chapter, log on to the PCOSA national website at: http://www.pcosupport.org. If you do not have access to the Internet, their postal address is:

Polycystic Ovarian Syndrome Association
PO Box 3403
Englewood, CO 80111

Through the ongoing efforts and partnership of physicians, researchers, and patients, Polycystic Ovary Syndrome will continue to become less of a mystery. Today the goals of fertility and good health are now within closer reach than ever for you.

Jill says, "It's a fascinating syndrome, so complicated. PCOS affects every woman differently and I don't think I will ever fully understand it, but this syndrome has changed my life! I am now more vigilant about my health and I will be even more vigilant of my daughter's health too! I have a more deep and meaningful respect for life. It is amazing how much your opinions change once you are faced with a health problem that you have little control over.

> This syndrome needs more public awareness and the more women and men who get involved in bringing PCOS to the public's attention, the more success we will have. Some words of wisdom to all women with PCOS out there is to love yourselves for who you are, please don't let this syndrome get you down. Fight back!

USEFUL WEBSITES

Polycystic Ovarian Syndrome Association- http://www. pcosupport.org

Soul Cysters, which looks at all aspects of PCOS and includes a free message board- http://www.soulcysters. com

16. RESOURCES -
Books, Glossary, Internet sites

BOOKS

Hart, Cheryle R. and Mary Kay Grossman, *The Insulin Resistance Diet--Revised and   updated* (McGraw-Hill, 2007)

Jonas, Steven and Linda Konner, *Just the Weigh You Are: How to be Fit and Healthy, Whatever Your Size* (Houghton Mifflin, 1998)

Legro, Richard S., Angela Boss and Evelina Weidman Sterling, *Living with P.C.O.S.:Polycystic Ovarian Syndrome* (Addicus Books, 2001)

Brand-Miller, Jennie, Thomas Wolever, Kaye Foster-Powell and Stephen Colagiuri *The New Glucose Revolution: The Authoritative Guide to the Glycemic Index - the Dietary Solution for Lifelong Health (Glucose Revolution)* (Marlowe & Company, 2006)

Steward, H. Leighton, Morrison Betha, Sam Andrews and Luis Balart, *The New Sugar Busters!* (Ballantine Books, 2003)

Harris, Colette and Adam Carey, *PCOS: A Woman's guide to Dealing with Polycystic Ovarian Syndrome* (Thorsons, 2000)

Thatcher, Samuel, *PCOS: The Hidden Epidemic* (Perspectives Press (IN), 2000)

Harris, Colette, *The PCOS Diet Book: How You Can Use the Nutritional Approach to Deal with Polycystic Ovary Syndrome* (Thorsons, 2002)

Rice, Rochelle, *Real Fitness for Real Women: A Unique Workout Program for the Plus-Size Woman* (Grand Central Publishing, 2001)

GLOSSARY

Clomid: The most commonly used fertility medication, given in tablet form. Also known as **Clomiphene.**

Dilatation and Curettage (D&C) - A minor surgical procedure in which the cervix is stretched slightly open and the internal lining of the uterus is sampled by scraping.

Glucophage - A commercial brand of metformin, an insulin sensitizing oral medication.

Hysterogram (hysterosalpingogram) - A radiologic procedure in which x-ray dye is injected into the uterus and fallopian tubes. Used to test for normality of the cavity of the uterus and whether the tubes are open or not.

Hysteroscopy (uteroscopy) - A minor surgical procedure in which a tubular-shaped scope is inserted through the cervix and into the uterus. Uses video to view the cavity and can also be used to operate through.

In vitro fertilization (IVF) - The most advanced fertility procedure available; eggs are removed from the ovaries, fertilized with the sperm in a lab dish, and the embryos transferred into the uterus.

Newborn/Neonatal Intensive Care Unit (NICU) - An intensive care unit for the critical care of premature and other critically ill newborns.

Ovarian drilling (Laparoscopic ovarian drilling (ovarian diathermy)) - A same day surgery procedure in which the surfaces or inside of the ovaries are burned or lasered in multiple locations. Used to treat infertility from PCOS. Watch a video of ovarian drilling at http://www.ivf.com/drilling.html.

INTERNET SITES- COMPLETE LIST

Advanced Fertility Center of Chicago- http://www.advancedfertility.com

The American Electrology Association- http://www.electrology.com

American Society for Reproductive Medicine- http://www.asrm.org

Androgen Excess and PCOS Society- www.androgenexcesssociety.org

The Atkins diet- http://atkins.com

Cedars Sinai where Dr. Ricardo Azziz works- http://www.cedars-sinai.edu

Center for PCOS at Drexel University College of Medicine- http://www.drexelmed.edu. Enter, "PCOS" in the website search box at top-right hand side of webpage.

This was the first multidisciplinary academic center for PCOS in the U.S.

DermNet NZ- http://www.dermnetnz.org/hair-nails-sweat/hirsutism.html

Doctors who are members of the Polycystic Ovarian Syndrome Association- http://www.pcosupport.org/membership/professionals.php

Dr. Shahab S. Minassian at The IVF-Fertility Program of the Women's Clinic, Ltd., Reading, PA.: www.infertilitypa.com. Click on the PCOS tab at the left of the home page.

HairFacts, an independent website dedicated to looking at how to control hair growth- http://www.hairfacts.com

Hair Removal- http://www.pcosupport.org/news/PCOSBulletin-June2005.pdf. (PCOS Bulletin. Volume 8, issue 1, June, 2005. Page 5).

Hirsutism report and PCOS with guides for managing hair growth. American Society for Reproductive Medicine-http://www.asrm.org/Patients/patientbooklets/hirsutismPCOS.pdf

Hirsutism medical and technical report- http://www.emedicine.com/derm/topic472.htm

The InterNational Council on Infertility Information Dissemination- www.inciid.org

The InterNational Council on Infertility Information Dissemination, Inc.- http://www.inciid.org

Jenny Craig, Inc.- http://www.jennycraig.com

Laser treatment- http://www.fda.gov/cdrh/consumer/laserfacts.html

Losing weight- http://www.soulcysters.com/weight_loss.html

http://www.weightloss.about.com/od/morediet1/a/
aa051005a.htm.

http://www.weightlossforall.com

Medical Terms- http://www.medterms.com/script/main/
hp.asp

The National Infertility Association- http://www.resolve.org

Polycystic Ovarian Syndrome Association- www.pcosupport.
org

RESOLVE: The National Infertility Association- www.
resolve.org

Slim-Fast- http://www.slim-fast.com

The Society of Reproductive Endocrinology and Infertility-
http://www.socrei.org

Soul Cysters- www.soulcysters.com

The South Beach Diet- http://www.southbeachdiet.com/
index3.asp

Sugar Busters- http://www.sugarbusters.com

Vaniqa- http://www.vaniqa.com

Various PCOS links from Georgia Reproductive Specialists-
http://www.ivf.com/links/pcoslinks.html

Vitaline- http://www.vitaline-slimming.com

Vitaline's PCOS website- http://www.vitaline-slimming.
com/pcos

Weight Watchers- http://www.weightwatchers.com

Endnotes

Chapter 1

[1] http://www.census.gov/population/socdemo/gender/ 2006gender_table1.1.csv. Information accessed on January 21, 2008.

[2] http://www.census.gov/ipc/www/idb- Click on "World Population Information" near the bottom, left-hand side of the page. This will bring up the following page:

http://www.census.gov/ipc/www/idb/worldpopinfo.html- Go near the bottom, left-hand side of the page where it reads, "World Population by Age and Sex", go to "select a year", select "2006" and click on "Submit Query."

The following webpage will come up- http://www.census.gov/ cgi-bin/ipc/idbagg

About the authors:

Christopher Hearn has a Journalism degree from Point Loma Nazarene University.

Shahab S. Minassian, M.D. is the Section Chief, Fertility and Reproductive Endocrinology at The Reading Hospital and Medical Center in Reading, PA. He is a staff physician with the IVF-Fertility Program at the Women's Clinic, Ltd. in Reading, PA. He also holds the title of Clinical Associate Professor of Obstetrics and Gynecology, Drexel University College of Medicine.